WEIGHT LOSS DIET RECIPES COOKBOOK

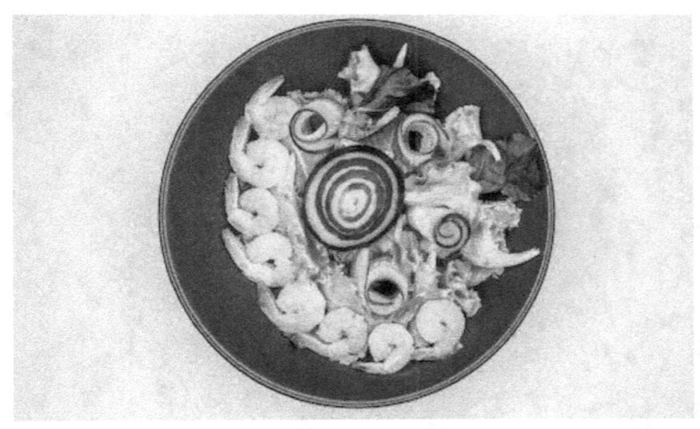

Dr. Kimberly Carlos

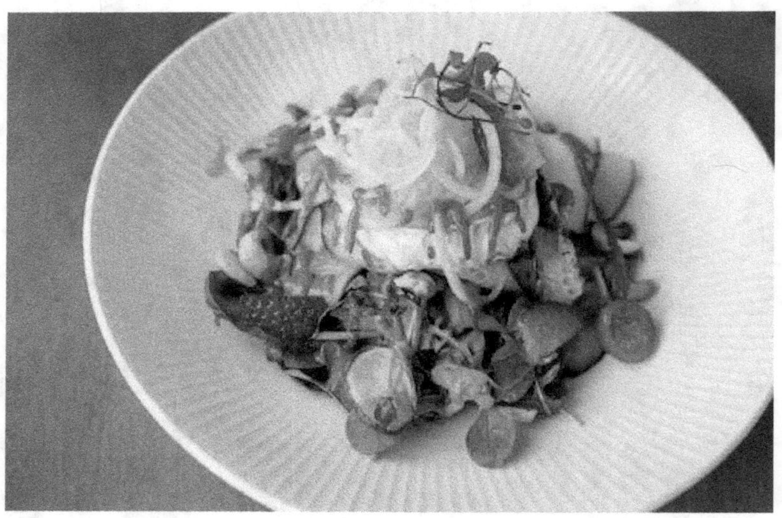

TABLE OF CONTENT

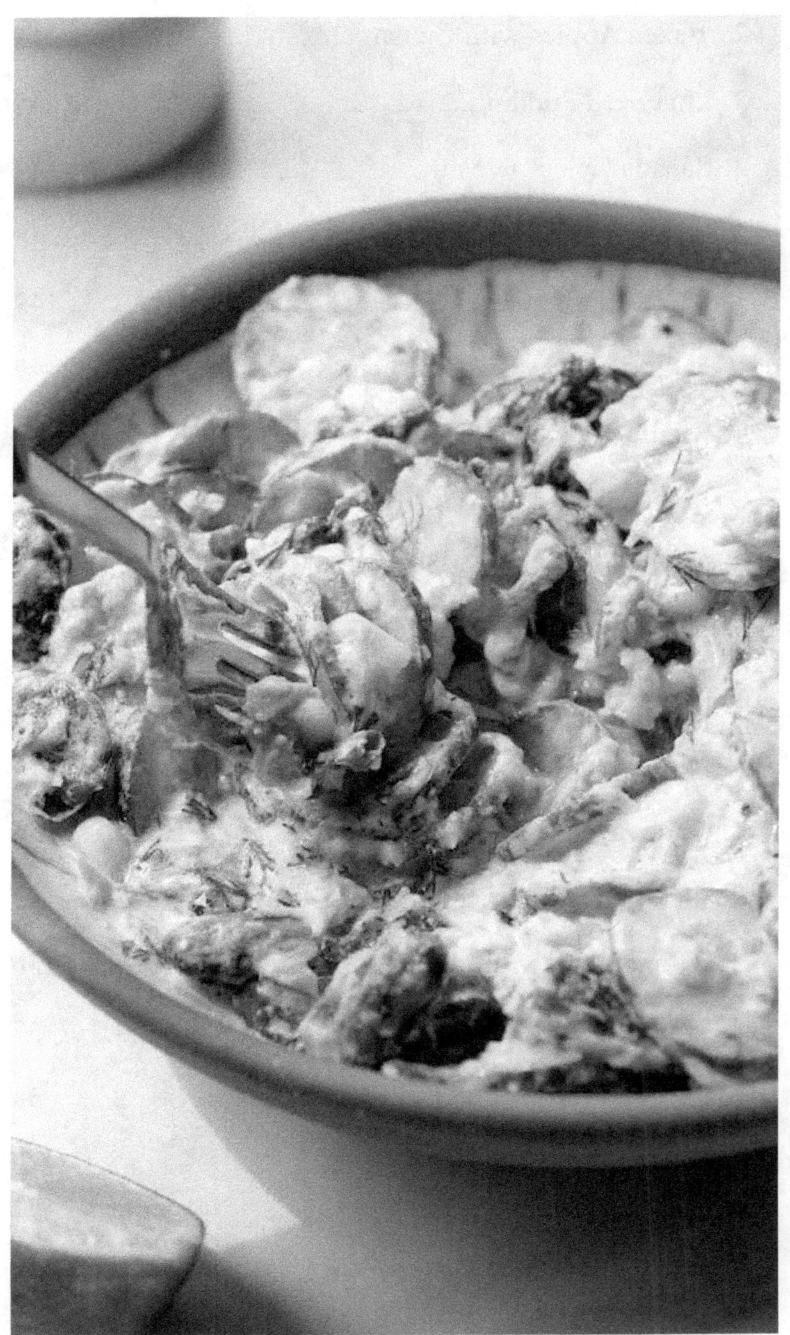

INTRODUCTION

Emily had always struggled with her weight. She had tried countless weight loss diets, only to be left disappointed and disheartened. However, this time was different. Determined to make a lasting change, she embarked on a new weight loss journey with unwavering determination.

Emily researched extensively and devised a well-balanced diet plan. She incorporated whole foods, vegetables, lean proteins, and healthy fats into her meals. She bid farewell to processed junk and embraced portion control. It was a challenging adjustment, but she remained resolute.

Every morning, Emily started her day with a nourishing breakfast—a bowl of oatmeal topped with fresh berries. For lunch, she enjoyed vibrant salads loaded with colorful vegetables and grilled chicken. Snack time meant a handful of nuts or a piece of fruit. Dinner was a delightful affair, with flavorful fish or chicken accompanied by steamed vegetables. She savored her meals and relished in the newfound energy they provided.

Emily complemented her diet with regular exercise. She hit the gym, joining various fitness classes that excited and motivated her. She discovered a passion for yoga and found solace in the practice, both physically and mentally. The endorphin rush she experienced became her driving force.

As the weeks passed, Emily noticed remarkable changes in her body and mind. Her clothes started fitting better, and she felt stronger and more confident. The weight on the scale decreased steadily, but more importantly, she felt healthier and happier than ever before.

Supportive friends and family rallied behind Emily, praising her dedication and progress. Their encouragement fueled her determination, making her believe in herself even more. She realized that this journey was about more than just weight loss—it was a testament to her strength and perseverance.

Months turned into a year, and Emily reached her weight loss goal. She had shed the extra pounds that had burdened her for so long. But this was just the beginning. Emily had discovered a new way of living—a lifestyle centered around nourishment, exercise, and self-care.

Inspired by her transformation, Emily decided to help others on their weight loss journeys. She became a certified nutritionist and established her practice, where she guided individuals towards sustainable and healthy habits. Her story served as a beacon of hope, reminding others that change was possible with dedication and a positive mindset.

Emily's weight loss diet had not only transformed her body but also her life. She was now living her passion, empowering others to embark on their own transformative journeys, and spreading the message of self-love and wellness to all who crossed her path.

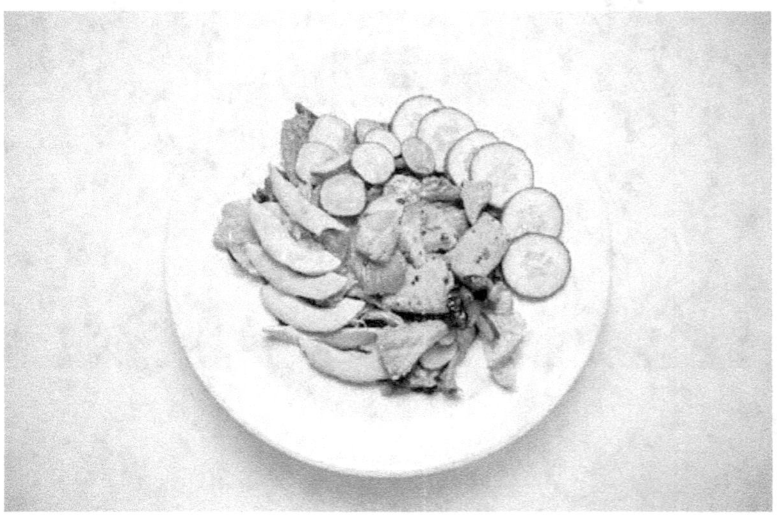

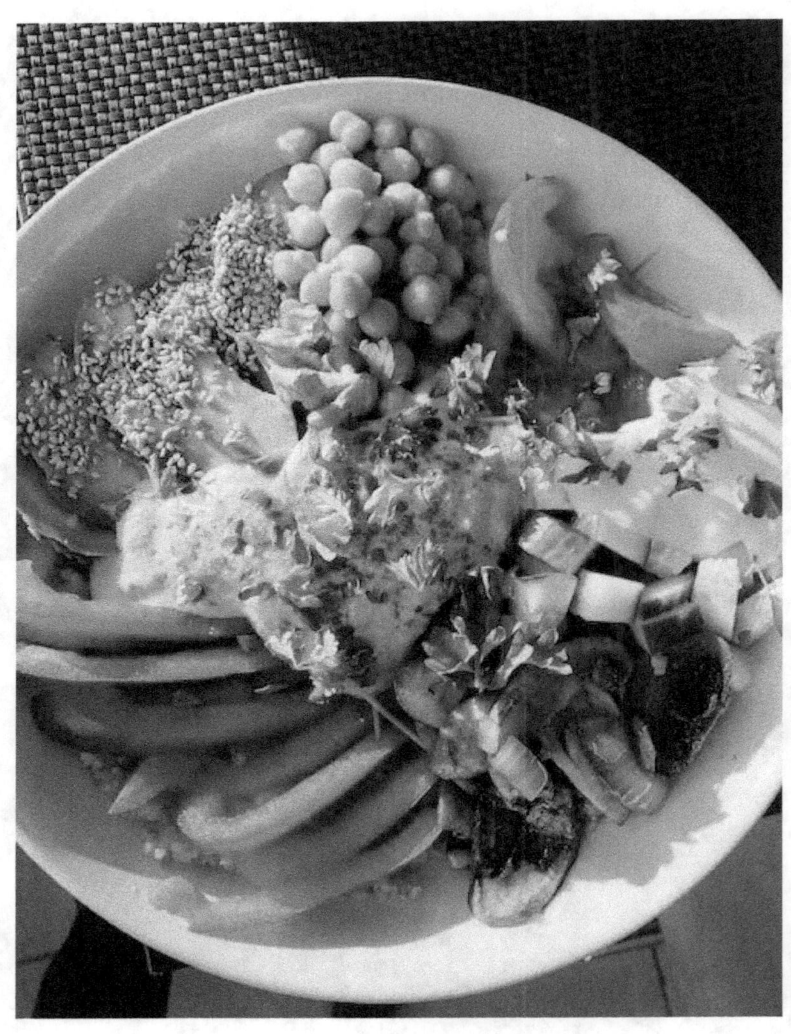

CHAPTER ONE

Weight Loss Diet and Benefits

In today's world, where sedentary lifestyles and unhealthy eating habits have become the norm, many individuals are seeking effective ways to achieve weight loss and improve their overall well-being.

A well-structured weight loss diet can be a powerful tool in achieving these goals. In this article, we will explore the benefits of following a weight loss diet and provide practical tips for success.

1. Sustainable Weight Loss

One of the primary benefits of a weight loss diet is achieving sustainable weight loss. By adopting a balanced and nutritious eating plan, you can create a calorie deficit while still meeting your body's nutritional needs. This approach encourages healthy, gradual weight loss, as opposed to crash diets that often lead to short-term results followed by weight regain. With a sustainable weight loss diet, you can establish lifelong habits that promote a healthy weight maintenance.

2. Improved Overall Health

Following a weight loss diet can lead to significant improvements in overall health. Obesity reduction can lower the risk of developing chronic conditions like diabetes, heart disease, and some types of cancer. A diet rich in fruits, vegetables, whole grains, lean proteins, and healthy fats provides essential nutrients, vitamins, and minerals that support optimal bodily functions. Additionally, losing weight can alleviate joint pain, improve sleep quality, enhance energy levels, and boost mood and self-confidence.

3. Increased Energy Levels

When you consume a well-balanced weight loss diet, your body receives the necessary fuel for optimal energy production. Whole foods rich in complex carbohydrates, such as whole grains, fruits, and vegetables, provide a steady release of energy throughout the day. By avoiding sugary, processed foods, you prevent energy crashes and maintain a consistent level of vitality. Regular physical activity, combined with a balanced diet, can further enhance your energy levels and improve overall fitness.

4. Enhanced Mental Well-being

The benefits of a weight loss diet extend beyond physical health. Research has shown a strong link between nutrition and mental well-being. Nutrient-dense foods can positively influence brain function and mood regulation. A diet rich in omega-3 fatty acids, found in fatty fish, nuts, and seeds, may help reduce symptoms of depression and anxiety. Additionally, consuming adequate vitamins and minerals, such as B vitamins and magnesium, supports optimal brain function and cognitive performance. By nourishing your body with wholesome foods, you can promote mental clarity, focus, and emotional stability.

5. Development of Healthy Eating Habits

Adopting a weight loss diet is an opportunity to cultivate healthy eating habits that can last a lifetime. By focusing on portion control, mindful eating, and the inclusion of nutrient-dense foods, you develop a better understanding of your body's nutritional needs. This awareness allows you to make informed food choices even after achieving your weight loss goals.

Over time, these healthy habits become second nature, leading to a sustainable lifestyle that supports long-term weight management and overall wellness.

Practical Tips for Following a Weight Loss Diet

1. Set realistic goals: Define achievable short-term and long-term goals that align with your overall health and well-being.

2. Seek professional guidance: Consult a registered dietitian or nutritionist to create a personalized weight loss plan tailored to your specific needs and preferences.

3. Plan your meals: Create a weekly meal plan that includes a variety of nutrient-dense foods. You'll be more organized and able to choose better options thanks to this.

4. Emphasize whole foods: Prioritize whole grains, lean proteins, fruits, vegetables, and healthy fats. Reduce your intake of processed meals, added sweets, and bad fats.

5. Practice portion control: Be mindful of portion sizes to maintain a calorie deficit while still meeting your nutritional needs. Use smaller portions and get comfortable recognizing your body's signals of hunger and fullness.

6. Stay hydrated: Drink an adequate amount of water throughout the day to support digestion, metabolism, and overall health.

7. Incorporate physical activity: Combine your weight loss diet with regular physical activity to maximize results, improve fitness levels, and promote overall well-being.

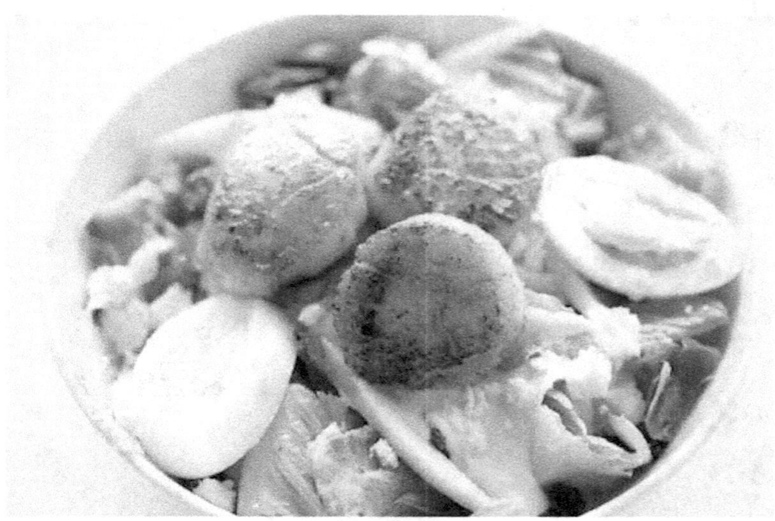

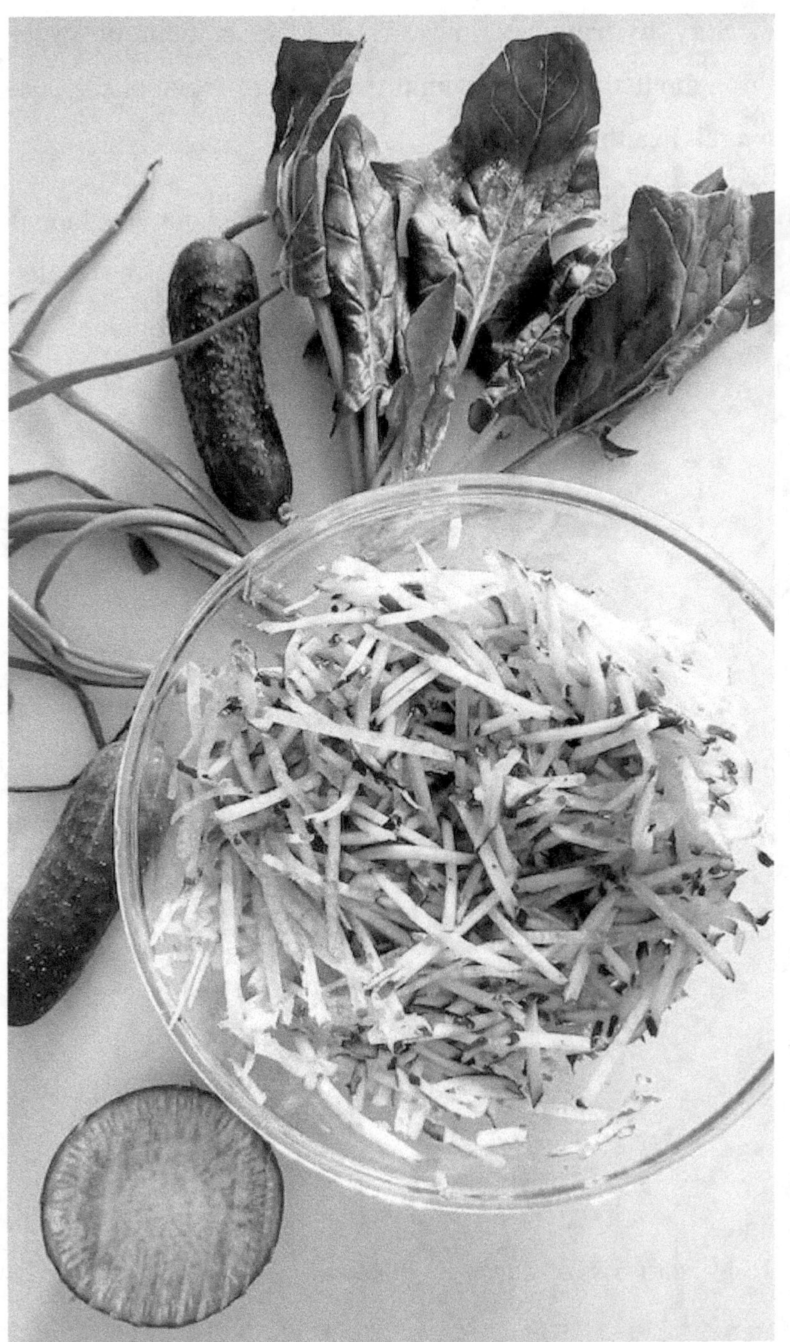

CHAPTER TWO

14 Day Weight Loss Diet Meal Plan

DAY 1

- Breakfast: Veggie omelet with spinach, bell peppers, and mushrooms.
- Snack: A small handful of almonds.
- Lunch: Grilled chicken breast with roasted vegetables.
- Snack: Greek yogurt with berries.
- Dinner: fish baked in the oven with quinoa and steam broccoli.

DAY 2

- Breakfast: Rolling oats, almond milk, chia seeds, and sliced fruit are combined to make overnight oats.
- Snack: Carrot sticks with hummus.
- Lunch: mixed greens, cherry tomatoes, cucumbers, and grilled shrimp in a quinoa salad.
- Snack: Apple slices with almond butter.
- Dinner: Grilled turkey breast with roasted Brussels sprouts and sweet potato.

DAY 3

- Breakfast: Whole wheat toast topped with avocado and a poached egg.
- Snack: Mixed berries.
- Lunch: Lentil soup with a side salad.
- Snack: Celery sticks with peanut butter.
- Dinner: Baked chicken breast with steamed asparagus and brown rice.

DAY 4

- Breakfast: Greek yogurt topped with banana slices and honey.
- Snack: Handful of walnuts.
- Lunch: Grilled tofu stir-fry with mixed vegetables.
- Snack: Orange slices.
- Dinner: fish baked with quinoa and roasted zucchini.

DAY 5

- Breakfast: Protein smoothie with spinach, a banana, almond milk, and a scoop of protein powder.
- Snack: Edamame beans.
- Lunch: Grilled chicken salad with mixed greens, cherry tomatoes, cucumber, and a light vinaigrette dressing.

- Snack: Cottage cheese with pineapple chunks.
- Dinner: Marinara sauce with zucchini noodles with turkey meatballs.

DAY 6

- Breakfast: Scrambled egg whites with sautéed spinach and cherry tomatoes.
- Snack: Grapefruit segments.
- Lunch: Quinoa-stuffed bell peppers.
- Snack: Rice cakes with almond butter.
- Dinner: Grilled shrimp skewers with grilled vegetables and quinoa.

DAY 7

- Breakfast: cereal made with whole grains, almond milk, and strawberry slices.
- Snack: Bell pepper slices with hummus.
- Lunch: Chickpea salad with mixed greens, cucumber, red onion, and a lemon vinaigrette dressing.
- Snack: Hard-boiled egg.
- Dinner: Grilled salmon with steamed asparagus and quinoa.

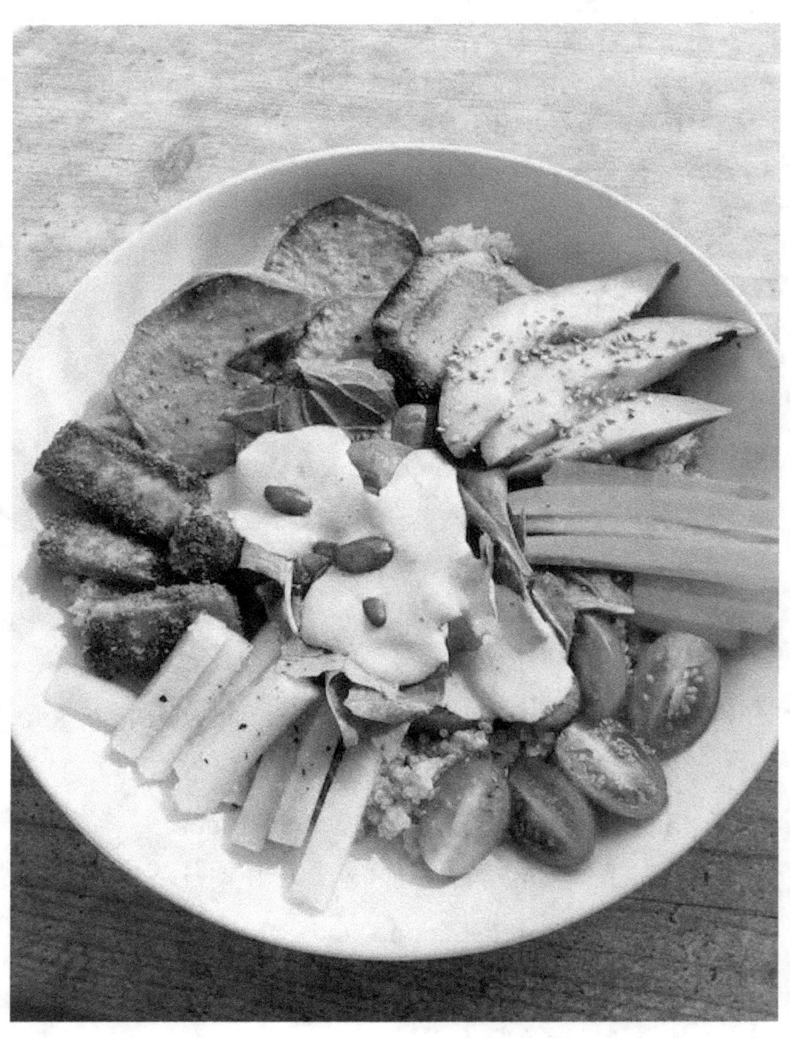

CHAPTER THREE

Weight Loss Diet Breakfast Recipes

1. Veggie Omelet

Start your day with a nutritious and protein-packed veggie omelet. Packed with vitamins and minerals from fresh vegetables, this recipe will keep you satisfied and energized throughout the morning.

Ingredients:

- 2 eggs
- 1/4 cup chopped spinach
- 1/4 cup diced bell peppers
- 1/4 cup sliced mushrooms
- Salt and pepper to taste
- 1 teaspoon olive oil

Instructions:

1. Beat the eggs in a bowl until fully combined. Add salt and pepper to taste.

2. In a nonstick skillet over medium heat, warm the olive oil.

3. Include the bell peppers, mushrooms, and spinach in the skillet. Sauté for 2 to 3 minutes or until softened somewhat.

4. Pour the beaten eggs on top of the skillet's vegetables.

5. Cook for 2-3 minutes or until the edges are set.

6. Carefully flip the omelet and cook for an additional 1-2 minutes.

7. Transfer to a plate and fold the omelet in half.

8. Serve hot and enjoy!

Cooking time: 10 minutes

2. Overnight Oats with Berries

This simple and delicious overnight oats recipe is perfect for busy mornings. Loaded with fiber, antioxidants, and healthy fats, it's a great way to kick-start your day.

Ingredients:

- 1/2 cup rolled oats
- 1/2 cup almond milk (or any other type of milk you want)
- 1 tbsp. chia seeds
- 1/2 cup blueberries, strawberries, and raspberries in a mixed-berry mixture
- 1 tablespoon honey (optional)

Instructions:

1. In a jar or container, combine rolled oats, almond milk, and chia seeds.

2. Be sure to thoroughly mix all the components.

3. Cover the jar/container and refrigerate overnight.

4. Stir the oats thoroughly in the morning.

5. Top with mixed berries and drizzle with honey, if desired.

6. Enjoy cold or microwave for a few seconds to warm it up.

Cooking time: Overnight (5 minutes hands-on time)

3. Avocado Toast with Poached Egg

Avocado toast is a popular and nutritious breakfast choice. This recipe adds a poached egg for an extra protein boost, making it a satisfying and balanced morning meal.

Ingredients:

- 1 slice whole wheat bread, toasted
- 1/2 ripe avocado, mashed
- 1 poached egg
- Salt and pepper to taste

Instructions:

1. Spread the mashed avocado evenly on the toasted bread.

2. Place the poached egg on top of the avocado.

3. Season to taste with salt and pepper.

4. Serve immediately.

Cooking time: 10 minutes

4. Protein Smoothie

A protein smoothie is a quick and convenient breakfast option, perfect for those on the go. Packed with protein and nutrients, it will keep you satisfied until lunchtime.

Ingredients:

- 1 cup almond milk, unsweetened (or any other milk of your choosing)
- 1 scoop of protein powder, in your choice of vanilla or another flavor.
- 1 handful of spinach
- 1 ripe banana
- Ice cubes (optional)

Instructions:

1. In a blender, combine almond milk, protein powder, spinach, and banana.

2. Blend until smooth and creamy.

3. If preferred, add ice cubes and mix one more.

4. Pour into a glass and start sipping right away.

Cooking time: 5 minutes

5. Greek Yogurt Parfait

This Greek yogurt parfait is a delightful and nutrient-rich breakfast option. Packed with protein, probiotics, and fiber, it's a refreshing way to start your day.

Ingredients:

- 1 cup Greek yogurt
- 1/4 cup granola
- 1/2 cup blueberries, strawberries, and raspberries in a mixed-berry mixture
- 1 tablespoon honey (optional)

Instructions:

1. Arrange Greek yogurt, granola, and mixed berries in a glass or bowl.

2. Drizzle with honey if desired.

3. Repeat the layers until all ingredients are used.

4. Top with a few extra berries.

5. Enjoy immediately.

Cooking time: 5 minutes

Weight Loss Diet Lunch Recipes

1. Grilled Chicken Salad

This grilled chicken salad is a satisfying and nutritious option for lunch. Packed with lean protein and colorful vegetables, it will keep you feeling full and energized throughout the day.

Ingredients:

- 4 oz grilled chicken breast, sliced
- 2 cups mixed salad greens
- 1/4 cup cherry tomatoes, halved

- 1/4 cup cucumber, sliced

- 1/4 cup red onion, thinly sliced

- 1 tablespoon balsamic vinaigrette dressing

Instructions:

1. In a large bowl, combine the mixed salad greens, cherry tomatoes, cucumber, and red onion.

2. Top the salad with the sliced grilled chicken breast.

3. Drizzle the balsamic vinaigrette dressing over the salad.

4. Toss gently to coat all ingredients.

5. Serve immediately.

Cooking time: 15 minutes (if chicken is pre-cooked)

2. Lentil Soup

A nourishing and comfortable lunch choice is lentil soup. Packed with fiber and plant-based protein, it's a satisfying meal that will keep you feeling full for hours.

Ingredients:

- 1 cup rinsed and drained dried lentils

-    1 carrot, diced

-    1 celery stalk, diced

-    1/2 onion, diced

-    2 garlic cloves, minced

-    4 cups vegetable broth

-    1 bay leaf

-    1 teaspoon cumin

-    Salt and pepper to taste

Instructions:

1. Warm up a small amount of oil in a big pot over medium heat.

2. Include the minced garlic, carrot, celery, and onion, all chopped. Vegetables should be sautéed for 5 minutes to soften.

3. Add the lentils, vegetable broth, bay leaf, cumin, salt, and pepper to the pot.

4. Bring the mixture to a boil, then reduce heat and simmer for 20-25 minutes or until lentils are tender.

5. Remove the bay leaf.

6. Use an immersion blender or blend half the soup in a regular blender until smooth (optional for a creamier texture).

7. Serve hot.

Cooking time: 30-35 minutes

3. Quinoa Salad

A versatile and wholesome lunch option is quinoa salad. Packed with plant-based protein, fiber, and a variety of vegetables, it's a satisfying and flavorful dish.

Ingredients:

- 1 cup cooked quinoa
- 1/2 cup cherry tomatoes, halved
- 1/2 cup cucumber, diced
- 1/4 cup red onion, thinly sliced
- 1/4 cup Kalamata olives, sliced
- 2 tablespoons feta cheese, crumbled
- 1 tablespoon lemon juice
- 1 tablespoon olive oil
- Salt and pepper to taste

Instructions:

1. Combine the cooked quinoa, Kalamata olives, feta cheese, cucumber, red onion, and cherry tomatoes in a big bowl.

2. To make the dressing, combine the lemon juice, olive oil, salt, and pepper in a separate small bowl.

3. Drizzle the quinoa salad with the dressing and gently toss to mix.

4. Serve chilled or at room temperature.

Cooking time: 20 minutes (if quinoa is pre-cooked)

4. Chickpea Salad Wrap

This chickpea salad wrap is a satisfying and flavorful lunch option. Packed with plant-based protein, fiber, and fresh vegetables, it's a healthy alternative to traditional sandwiches.

Ingredients:

- 1 cup washed and drained canned chickpeas
- 1/4 cup diced cucumber
- 1/4 cup diced bell peppers

- 2 tablespoons diced red onion

- 2 tablespoons chopped fresh parsley

- 1 tablespoon lemon juice

- 1 tablespoon olive oil

- Salt and pepper to taste

- Whole grain wraps or lettuce leaves for serving

Instructions:

1. In a medium bowl, mash the chickpeas using a fork or potato masher until they reach a chunky consistency.

2. Add the diced cucumber, bell peppers, red onion, parsley, lemon juice, olive oil, salt, and pepper to the bowl. Stir well to combine.

3. Taste and adjust seasoning if needed.

4. Scoop the chickpea salad onto whole grain wraps or lettuce leaves.

5. Roll up the wraps or fold the lettuce leaves around the salad.

6. Serve immediately.

Cooking time: 10 minutes

5. Grilled Tofu Stir-Fry

This grilled tofu stir-fry is a delicious and nutritious lunch option for vegetarians or those looking to incorporate more plant-based meals. Packed with protein and colorful vegetables, it's a flavorful and satisfying dish.

Ingredients:

- 8 oz firm tofu, pressed and cut into cubes
- 2 cups mixed vegetables (such as bell peppers, broccoli, snap peas)
- 2 tablespoons low-sodium soy sauce
- 1 tablespoon sesame oil
- 1 garlic clove, minced
- 1 teaspoon grated ginger
- 1/4 teaspoon red pepper flakes (optional)
- Salt and pepper to taste

Instructions:

1. In a small bowl, whisk together the soy sauce, sesame oil, minced garlic, grated ginger, red pepper flakes (if using), salt, and pepper.

2. Preheat a grill pan or non-stick skillet over medium-high heat.

3. Grill the tofu cubes for 3-4 minutes on each side until lightly browned.

4. Take the tofu out of the skillet and place it aside.

5. In the same pan, add the mixed vegetables and stir-fry for 5-6 minutes until crisp-tender.

6. Return the grilled tofu to the pan and pour the sauce over the tofu and vegetables.

7. Stir-fry for an additional 2 minutes to heat everything through and coat with the sauce.

8. Serve hot.

Cooking time: 20 minutes

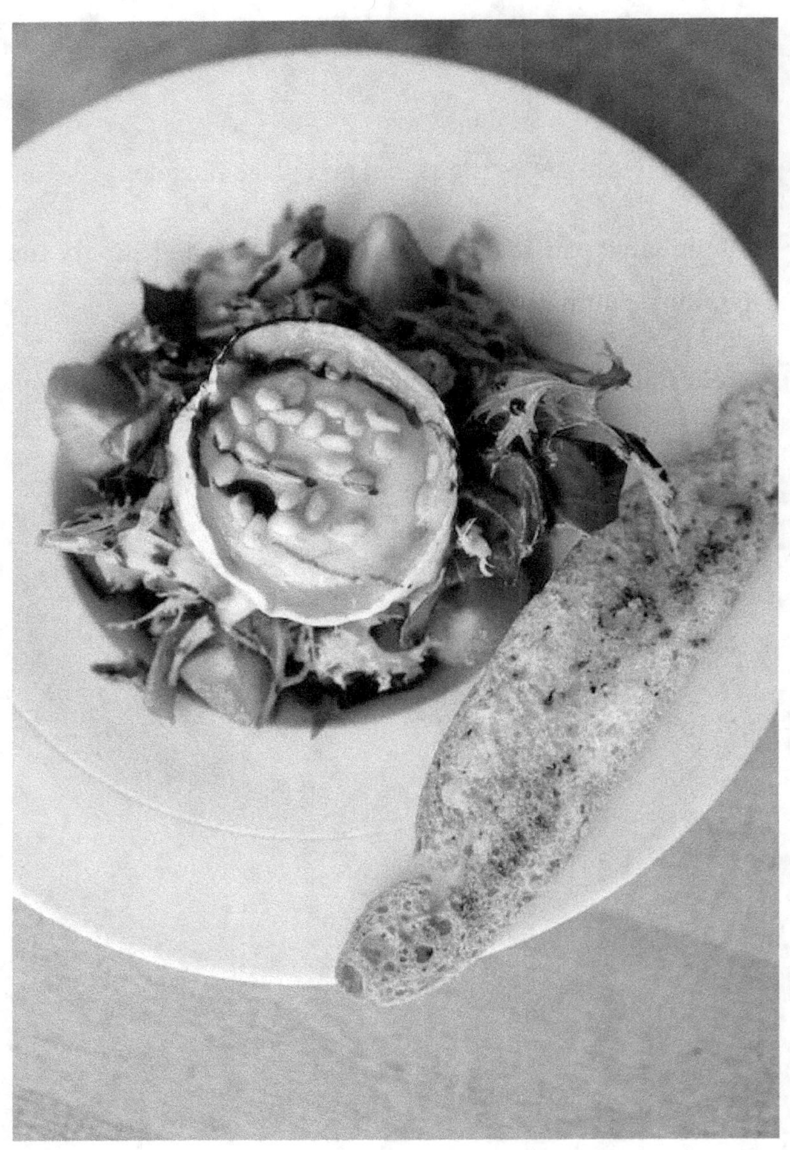

CHAPTER FOUR

Weight Loss Diet Dinner Recipes

1. Baked Salmon with Roasted Vegetables

Served with roasted veggies, this baked salmon dish makes a filling and tasty evening. Packed with heart-healthy omega-3 fatty acids and an array of colorful vegetables, it's a well-rounded meal for weight loss.

Ingredients:

- 4 oz salmon fillet
- 1 cup of mixed vegetables, including carrots, bell peppers, and broccoli
- 1 tablespoon olive oil
- 1 teaspoon lemon juice
- Salt and pepper to taste

Instructions:

1. Set the oven's temperature to 400°F (200°C).

2. Arrange the salmon fillet on a parchment-lined baking pan.

3. Combine the olive oil, lemon juice, salt, and pepper in a

small bowl.

4. Brush the olive oil mixture over the salmon fillet.

5. Arrange the mixed vegetables around the salmon on the baking sheet.

6. Drizzle the vegetables with a little olive oil and season with salt and pepper.

7. Bake for 15 to 18 minutes in a preheated oven, or until the salmon is cooked through and the veggies are soft.

8. Serve hot.

Cooking time: 20-25 minutes

2. Turkey Meatballs with Zucchini Noodles

These turkey meatballs with zucchini noodles are a healthy and low-carb alternative to traditional pasta dishes. Packed with lean protein and fiber, it's a satisfying and delicious dinner option.

Ingredients:

- 4 oz ground turkey
- 1/4 cup whole wheat breadcrumbs

- 1/4 cup grated Parmesan cheese

- 1 egg, beaten

- 1 garlic clove, minced

- 1/4 teaspoon dried oregano

- Salt and pepper to taste

- 2 medium zucchini, sliced into noodles or spirals

- 1 cup marinara sauce

Instructions:

1. In a large bowl, combine ground turkey, breadcrumbs, Parmesan cheese, beaten egg, minced garlic, dried oregano, salt, and pepper. Mix well.

2. Shape the mixture into small meatballs.

3. Preheat a non-stick skillet over medium heat and lightly coat with cooking spray.

4. Cook the turkey meatballs in the skillet for 8-10 minutes, turning occasionally, until cooked through and browned.

5. In a separate large skillet, heat the marinara sauce over medium heat.

6. Add the zucchini noodles to the skillet and cook for 3-4 minutes until slightly softened.

7. Divide the zucchini noodles among plates and top with the turkey meatballs.

8. Serve hot.

Cooking time: 25-30 minutes

3. Lentil Curry with Brown Rice

This lentil curry with brown rice is a flavorful and nutritious dinner option. Packed with plant-based protein, fiber, and aromatic spices, it's a satisfying meal for weight loss.

Ingredients:

- 1 cup dried red lentils
- 1 cup diced tomatoes
- 1 small onion, diced
- 2 garlic cloves, minced
- 1 tablespoon curry powder
- 1 teaspoon ground cumin
- 1/2 teaspoon turmeric powder
- 1/4 teaspoon cayenne pepper (optional)
- 2 cups vegetable broth
- Salt and pepper to taste
- Cooked brown rice for serving
- Chopped fresh cilantro for garnish (optional)

Instructions:

1. Rinse the red lentils under cold water and drain.

2. In a large pot, sauté the diced onion and minced garlic over medium heat until softened.

3. Include the cayenne pepper (if using), curry powder, ground cumin, turmeric powder, and ground cumin. To evenly coat the onions and garlic, stir thoroughly.

4. Fill the container with the red lentils, vegetable broth, and diced tomatoes. Add salt and pepper to taste.

5. After bringing the mixture to a boil, lower the heat to a simmer and cook the mixture for 20 to 25 minutes, or until the lentils are soft and the curry has thickened.

6. Spoon the cooked brown rice over the lentil curry.

7. If preferred, garnish with finely chopped fresh cilantro.

Cooking time: 30-35 minutes

4. Grilled Chicken Breast with Steamed Asparagus and Quinoa

This grilled chicken breast with steamed asparagus and quinoa is a well-balanced and satisfying dinner option. Packed with lean protein, fiber, and nutrients, it's a wholesome meal for weight loss.

Ingredients:

- 4 oz chicken breast
- 1 cup asparagus spears, trimmed
- 1/2 cup cooked quinoa
- 1 tablespoon lemon juice
- 1 tablespoon olive oil
- Salt and pepper to taste

Instructions:

1. Turn on the medium-high heat and prepare a grill or grill pan.
2. Add salt, pepper, lemon juice, and olive oil to the chicken breast to season it.
3. Cook the chicken breast on the grill for 6 to 8 minutes on each side.

4. Steam the asparagus spears for 4-5 minutes, or until crisp-tender, while the chicken is roasting.

5. After the chicken has finished cooking, take it off the grill and give it a moment to rest before slicing.

6. Serve the grilled chicken breast with steamed asparagus and cooked quinoa.

7. Drizzle with additional lemon juice if desired.

8. Serve hot.

Cooking time: 20-25 minutes

5. Baked Cod with Roasted Brussels Sprouts and Sweet Potato

This baked cod with roasted Brussels sprouts and sweet potato is a flavorful and nutritious dinner option. Packed with omega-3 fatty acids, vitamins, and fiber, it's a well-rounded meal for weight loss.

Ingredients:

- 4 oz cod fillet
- 1 cup halved and trimmed Brussels sprouts
- 1 tiny sweet potato, diced after being peeled
- 1 tablespoon olive oil

- 1/2 teaspoon paprika
- Salt and pepper to taste
- Lemon wedges for serving

Instructions:

1. Preheat the oven to 400°F (200°C).
2. Place the cod fillet on a baking sheet lined with parchment paper.
3. In a separate bowl, combine the Brussels sprouts, sweet potato cubes, olive oil, paprika, salt, and pepper. Toss to coat the vegetables evenly.
4. Arrange the Brussels sprouts and sweet potato around the cod on the baking sheet.
5. Bake in the preheated oven for 15-18 minutes, or until the cod is cooked through and the vegetables are tender.
6. Serve the baked cod with roasted Brussels sprouts and sweet potato.
7. Squeeze fresh lemon juice over the cod fillet before serving.
8. Serve hot.

Cooking time: 25-30 minutes

Weight Loss Diet Dessert Recipes

1. Greek Yogurt Parfait with Berries

This Greek yogurt parfait with berries is a light and satisfying dessert option. Packed with protein, calcium, and antioxidants, it's a guilt-free treat that will satisfy your sweet tooth.

Ingredients:

- 1 cup Greek yogurt
- 1/4 cup granola
- 1/2 cup blueberries, strawberries, and raspberries in a mixed-berry mixture
- 1 tablespoon honey (optional)

Instructions:

1. Arrange Greek yogurt, granola, and mixed berries in a glass or bowl.
2. Drizzle with honey if desired.
3. Repeat the layers until all ingredients are used.
4. Serve chilled.

Preparation time: 5 minutes

2. Baked Apples with Cinnamon

These baked apples with cinnamon are a warm and comforting dessert option. Packed with fiber and natural sweetness, they provide a healthy alternative to traditional baked goods.

Ingredients:

- 2 apples
- 1 tablespoon lemon juice
- 1 tablespoon honey
- 1/2 teaspoon cinnamon

Instructions:

1. Preheat the oven to 375°F (190°C).

2. Core the apples and remove the seeds, creating a hollow center.

3. Place the apples in a baking dish and drizzle with lemon juice.

4. Drizzle honey over the apples and sprinkle with cinnamon.

5. Bake in the preheated oven for 25-30 minutes, or until the apples are tender.

6. Take them out of the oven and allow them to cool a bit before serving.

7. Enjoy warm.

Cooking time: 25-30 minutes

3. Chia Seed Pudding

Chia seed pudding is a nutritious and versatile dessert option. Packed with omega-3 fatty acids, fiber, and antioxidants, it's a satisfying treat that can be customized with various flavors and toppings.

Ingredients:

- 2 tablespoons chia seeds
- 1 cup almond milk, unsweetened (or any other milk of your choosing)
- 1 tablespoon maple syrup (optional)
- 1/2 teaspoon vanilla extract
- Toppings of your choice (e.g., fresh fruits, nuts, shredded coconut)

Instructions:

1. Combine the chia seeds, almond milk, vanilla extract, and maple syrup (if using) in a bowl.

2. Stir thoroughly to distribute the chia seeds evenly.

3. After 10 minutes, stir the mixture once more to remove any clumps.

4. Once the mixture has thickened and taken on the consistency of pudding, cover the bowl and chill for at least two hours or overnight.

5. Stir well before serving and adjust the sweetness if desired.

6. Top with your favorite fruits, nuts, or shredded coconut.

7. Serve chilled.

Preparation time: 5 minutes + refrigeration time

4. Banana "Nice" Cream

Banana "Nice" Cream is a creamy and delicious frozen dessert option without the added sugars and fats found in traditional ice cream. It's a simple and healthy treat that can be enjoyed guilt-free.

Ingredients:

- 2 ripe bananas, peeled and frozen
- 1-2 tablespoons almond milk (or any milk of your choice)
- Toppings of your choice (e.g., dark chocolate chips, chopped nuts, sliced fruits)

Instructions:

1. Place the frozen bananas in a blender or food processor.
2. Blend until creamy and smooth after adding 1 tablespoon of almond milk. If extra milk is required, add it to get the right consistency.
3. Transfer the banana "nice" cream to a bowl.
4. Add your favorite toppings such as dark chocolate chips, chopped nuts, or sliced fruits.
5. Serve immediately.

Preparation time: 5 minutes

5. Mixed Berry Salad

A mixed berry salad is a refreshing and naturally sweet dessert option. Packed with antioxidants, vitamins, and fiber, it's a healthy and light choice for satisfying your sweet cravings.

Ingredients:

- 1 cup of mixed berries, including blackberries, raspberries, blueberries, and strawberries.
- Fresh mint leaves for garnish
- 1 tablespoon honey or a drizzle of balsamic glaze (optional)

Instructions:

1. Rinse the mixed berries under cold water and drain.
2. Place the mixed berries in a bowl.
3. Garnish with fresh mint leaves.
4. Drizzle with honey or balsamic glaze if desired.
5. Toss gently to combine.
6. Serve chilled.

Preparation time: 5 minutes

CHAPTER FIVE

Weight Loss Diet Snacks Recipes

1. Veggie Sticks with Hummus

This veggie sticks with hummus recipe is a nutritious and satisfying snack option. Packed with fiber, vitamins, and healthy fats, it's a great way to incorporate more vegetables into your diet.

Ingredients:

- Mixed vegetable sticks (cucumber, bell peppers, carrots, celery)
- Hummus for dipping

Instructions:

1. Wash the vegetables and chop them into sticks.

2. Arrange the vegetable sticks on a plate.

3. Serve with a side of hummus for dipping.

4. Enjoy!

Preparation time: 10 minutes

2. Greek Yogurt with Berries

Greek yogurt with berries is a protein-rich and antioxidant-packed snack option. It's quick to prepare and makes for a refreshing and satisfying treat.

Ingredients:

- 1 cup Greek yogurt
- 1/2 cup blueberries, strawberries, and raspberries in a mixed-berry mixture
- 1 tablespoon honey (optional)

Instructions:

1. In a bowl or cup, scoop the Greek yogurt.

2. Top with mixed berries.

3. Drizzle with honey, if desired.

4. Mix gently to combine.

5. Enjoy!

Preparation time: 5 minutes

3. Hard-Boiled Eggs with Avocado

Hard-boiled eggs with avocado is a protein-rich and healthy fat-filled snack option. It provides a good balance of nutrients and keeps you feeling satisfied between meals.

Ingredients:

- 2 hard-boiled eggs
- 1/2 avocado, sliced
- Salt and pepper to taste

Instructions:

1. Cut the hard-boiled eggs in half after peeling them.

2. Arrange the egg halves on a plate.

3. Top each egg half with avocado slices.

4. Season to taste with salt and pepper.

5. Enjoy!

Preparation time: 10 minutes (if hard-boiled eggs are pre-cooked)

4. Trail Mix

A versatile and portable food choice is trail mix. Packed with a variety of nuts, seeds, and dried fruits, it provides a good balance of protein, healthy fats, and fiber.

Ingredients:

- 1/2 cup almonds
- 1/4 cup walnuts
- 1/4 cup pumpkin seeds
- 1/4 cup dried cranberries
- 1/4 cup unsweetened coconut flakes

Instructions:

1. Combine all the ingredients in a bowl.

2. Toss well to mix evenly.

3. Transfer the trail mix to a resealable container or portion into individual snack bags.

4. Enjoy as a grab-and-go snack!

Preparation time: 5 minutes

5. Rice Cakes with Almond Butter and Banana Slices

Rice cakes with almond butter and banana slices make for a simple, satisfying, and energizing snack option. They provide a combination of carbohydrates, healthy fats, and natural sweetness.

Ingredients:

- Rice cakes
- Almond butter
- Banana, thinly sliced

Instructions:

1. Spread a thin layer of almond butter onto each rice cake.

2. Arrange banana slices on top of the almond butter.

3. Serve and enjoy!

Preparation time: 5 minutes

Weight Loss Diet Smoothies and Juicing Recipes

1. Green Detox Smoothie

This green detox smoothie is packed with nutrient-rich ingredients that support detoxification and weight loss. It's a tasty and revitalizing way to start the day.

Ingredients:

- 1 cup spinach
- 1/2 cup cucumber, chopped
- 1/2 green apple, chopped
- 1/2 lemon, juiced
- 1/2 inch ginger, grated
- 1 cup coconut water
- Ice cubes (optional)

Instructions:

1. Fill a blender with all the ingredients.
2. Blend until creamy and smooth.
3. Reblender after adding ice cubes, if preferred.
4. Pour into a glass and start sipping right away.

Preparation time: 5 minutes

2. Berry Blast Smoothie

This berry blast smoothie is a delicious and antioxidant-rich option for weight loss. Packed with berries and greens, it provides a burst of vitamins and minerals.

Ingredients:

- Blueberries, strawberries, and raspberries make up one cup of mixed berries.
- 1/2 cup baby kale or spinach
- 1/2 cup almond milk, unsweetened (or any other milk of your choosing)
- 1 tbsp. chia seeds
- Optional: 1 teaspoon honey or maple syrup
- Ice cubes (optional)

Instructions:

1. Fill a blender with all the ingredients.
2. Blend until creamy and smooth.
3. Reblender after adding ice cubes, if preferred.
4. Pour into a glass and start sipping right away.

Preparation time: 5 minutes

3. Tropical Green Juice

This tropical green juice is a refreshing and hydrating option that combines the sweetness of tropical fruits with the goodness of leafy greens.

Ingredients:

- 1 cup spinach
- 1/2 cup chopped pineapple
- 1/2 cup chopped mango
- 1/2 cucumber, chopped
- 1/2 lime, juiced
- 1/2 cup coconut water
- Ice cubes (optional)

Instructions:

1. Place all the ingredients in a juicer.

2. Process until all the ingredients are juiced.

3. Reblender after adding ice cubes, if preferred.

4. Pour into a glass and start sipping right away.

Preparation time: 5 minutes

4. Protein-Packed Chocolate Smoothie

This protein-packed chocolate smoothie is a satisfying and indulgent option for weight loss. It provides a good balance of protein, healthy fats, and natural sweetness.

Ingredients:

- 1 cup almond milk, unsweetened (or any other milk of your choosing)
- 1 scoop chocolate protein powder
- 1 tablespoon unsweetened cocoa powder
- 1/2 frozen banana
- 1 tablespoon almond butter
- Ice cubes (optional)

Instructions:

1. Fill a blender with all the ingredients.

2. Blend until creamy and smooth.

3. Reblender after adding ice cubes, if preferred.

4. Pour into a glass and start sipping right away

Preparation time: 5 minutes

5. Beet and Carrot Juice

This beet and carrot juice is a vibrant and nutrient-dense option that supports detoxification and weight loss. It's a flavorful way to incorporate more vegetables into your diet.

Ingredients:

- 1 medium beet, peeled and chopped
- 2 medium carrots, peeled and chopped
- 1 apple, chopped
- 1/2 lemon, juiced
- 1-inch ginger, grated
- Ice cubes (optional)

Instructions:

1. Place all the ingredients in a juicer.

2. Process until all the ingredients are juiced.

3. Reblender after adding ice cubes, if preferred.

4. Pour into a glass and start sipping right away.

Preparation time: 5 minutes

CONCLUSION

In conclusion, a weight loss diet is a valuable tool for individuals aiming to shed excess pounds and improve their overall health and well-being.

While there is no one-size-fits-all approach to weight loss, incorporating key principles and making mindful choices can lead to successful and sustainable results.

A weight loss diet emphasizes the importance of consuming nutrient-dense foods while reducing calorie intake. By choosing whole, unprocessed foods and incorporating a variety of fruits, vegetables, lean proteins, whole grains, and healthy fats, individuals can nourish their bodies while promoting weight loss.

These food choices provide essential vitamins, minerals, fiber, and antioxidants, which support overall health and help to curb cravings.

Portion control is a critical aspect of a weight loss diet. By practicing mindful eating and being aware of portion sizes, individuals can create a calorie deficit without feeling deprived.

Eating slowly, savoring each bite, and listening to hunger and fullness cues can contribute to a healthier relationship with food and prevent overeating.

Another crucial element of a weight loss program is regular exercise. Combining a balanced diet with exercise helps to boost metabolism, increase calorie burn, preserve muscle mass, and promote overall fitness.

Incorporating a mix of cardiovascular exercises, strength training, and flexibility exercises can lead to optimal results and enhance overall well-being.

While weight loss diets typically focus on reducing calorie intake, it's important to prioritize nutrient density and the overall quality of the diet. Crash diets or extreme calorie restriction can lead to nutrient deficiencies and other health issues.

Therefore, it is crucial to consult with a healthcare professional or registered dietitian to develop a personalized weight loss plan that meets individual nutritional needs and preferences.

When starting a weight loss program, consistency and patience are essential. Sustainable weight loss takes time and requires long-term commitment. It's important to approach weight loss with a positive mindset, focusing on overall health and well-being rather than solely the number on the scale.

Celebrating non-scale victories, such as increased energy, improved mood, and better sleep, can help maintain motivation and sustain healthy habits.

It's worth noting that individual results may vary, and it's essential to listen to your body and make adjustments as needed. What works for one person may not work for another, so it's crucial to personalize your weight loss approach and find what suits you best.

Finally, a weight loss diet is not a one-time endeavor but rather a lifestyle change. Once weight loss goals are achieved, it's important to transition into a maintenance phase by adopting sustainable habits that promote weight maintenance and overall health.

This includes maintaining a balanced diet, staying physically active, managing stress levels, and seeking support from healthcare professionals, registered dietitians, or support groups if needed.

In conclusion, a weight loss diet can be an effective and sustainable approach to achieve weight loss and improve overall health.

By focusing on nutrient-dense foods, portion control, regular physical activity, and a positive mindset, individuals can create lasting change and embark on a journey towards a healthier and happier life.

Remember, it's not just about losing weight—it's about nurturing your body, embracing a balanced lifestyle, and taking care of yourself in the best possible way.